Home Doctor

Use Proven and Natural Recipes Made of Herbs To Prevent and Cure Illness

Table of Contents

Introduction

A natural healing remedy is all about effective healing which supports your body's best efforts at healing you. It's important that you do support your body in the healing process, rather than suppressing it, as this always makes for improved health in the long term.

Suppressing your symptoms may give you the impression that the problem has gone away, but in reality, it is still there, smoldering under the surface, waiting for an opportunity to appear again.

By learning how to use the common homeopathic remedies at home, you can support your immune system, saving yourself a lot of money, time and improve your health both in the short and long term.

Homeopathy is a complete and natural system of health care which is as able to successfully treat the complex and serious disease as it can treat minor problems. It treats both physical and emotional imbalances. And it's also flexible in its approach. You can visit a professional homeopath for all your health needs, and you can learn to use some common remedies yourself.

There are many homeopathic home prescribing remedies which you can learn to use without a great deal of knowledge.

First, you need to buy a homeopathic home prescribing kit. This is by far the most economical way of buying homeopathic remedies. It also means that you have immediate access to many of the common remedies you will find you need on a day to day basis.

Make sure you buy your kit from a reputable homeopath or homeopathic pharmacy.

Then you need to read the instructions thoroughly. Homeopathy is different from any other modality of health care, so it can take time to get your head around the principles.

Next, you need to find some classes to attend, either in person or on the internet. The importance of classes should never be under-estimated. They can speed up your learning process, provide a sharing experience with other students and the teacher should be available for your problems.

Once you know how to use the common homeopathic home prescribing remedies, you'll wonder how you ever managed without them.

Chapter 1: Natural Healing Remedies

In any capitalistic, western society there are always going to be resentments and protests towards any form of healthcare other than traditional western medicine. Anyone in pursuit of a more natural approach towards healthcare to cure their ailments will soon understand this, as the waves of criticism come from friends, family, and so-called experts in medicine. To a certain degree, these criticisms are not unfounded at least to the point of raising concern. It is an actual system of checks and balances within the western private healthcare system that these issues perpetuate and eliminate any chance of medical professionals in western society to endorse any of the natural healing remedies publicly.

This method has to have special features to suppress any naturopathic healing within a society organically:

1) healthcare has to be controlled by private industry

2) western medicine is the dominating field of healthcare and

3) to put bluntly, it has to be a legally conscious society that has a propensity to sue such as the U.S.A.

Private pharmaceutical companies develop new drugs that improve symptoms of a particular illness. Those same companies establish incentive programs and provide kickbacks to private practitioners and other medical professions to use their products. These medical specialists and pharmaceutical companies are backed by top liability insurance policies, massive legal departments, and a large cushion of assets.

Eventually, one of these magic pills these pharmaceutical behemoths rush to the markets backfire. There was either not enough testing, MDs overprescribe or misprescribe a new drug, or patients wrongfully prescribe themselves-in any case this results in two possible outcomes an overwhelming response of negative side affects, including death, eliminates the drug from the market or a particular drug will remain on the market due to the fact that it is still profitable even after compensation to the injured parties or compensation to the families.

The bottom line western medicine drugs' successes are directly tied to the revenue generated. The higher the profit, the better the drug success (not its ability to combat particular symptoms) and thus we have our system.

Now, what does this have to due with natural healing remedies? Simple, western medicine drugs are designed to treat symptoms. Naturopathic healing, homeopathic medicine, eastern medicine, and many alternative medicines are designed to cure. THERE IS NO MONEY IN CURES, and therefore no room for natural healing remedies in western medicine.

What would a cure be to most private practitioners? An inflated one time charge or a remedy that is so simple it can be duplicated at home (in which case the exchange of money would be the cost of an office visit). If there is no money in cures, then there would be no money in any natural healing remedy. Thus these practices would never be endorsed by a medical professional in a society with a medical system similar to that of the US.

This is nothing new and is, for the most part, common knowledge, but people that live in such societies feel helpless and continue to choose western medicine over other forms of healthcare simply because it is the cultural norm as well as the fear of deviating from their "all knowing" doctor's opinion. Therefore it is imperative for all to arm themselves with the knowledge of various forms of healthcare and decide for themselves which is the correct path to healing.

Chapter 2: Migraines

Migraines are an extreme type of a headache that can completely prevent you from functioning normally. Characterized by photophobia, hypersensitivity to sounds and smells, as well and nausea and vomiting, you should not underestimate the severity of symptoms that a migraine can involve.

Special Anti-Migraine Herbal Blend

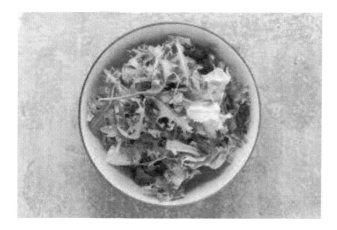

Ingredients: 50 grams of hops, bark viburnum reef, speedwell herb, lemon balm leaf, lavender flower, fruit fennel, sweet flag rhizome, St. John's wort, valerian root and flower primrose.

Mix a tablespoon of the above ingredients into a glass of boiling water and brew for 3 hours, covered.

Before consuming, gently heat the blend up. We recommend consuming the drink 15 minutes before a meal. The drink should be taken 3 times a day, with a fresh brew being prepared each time.

Amber Massage

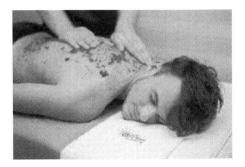

A tincture of amber massage can also assist in getting rid of a migraine. A tincture, or liquid extract of a herb, can be made by combining ¼ liter of spirits, and 50 grams of fine, natural amber. Leave this mixture in a closed container in a dark place for two weeks. Alternatively, you can purchase it from your local herb or health store.

Foot Spa

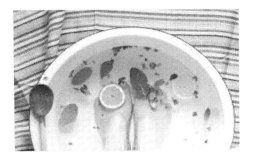

A great way to alleviate migraines is by having a foot bath.

Pour hot water into a bowl, tub, or bucket and add 4 drops of rosemary water. Soak your feet in hot water for around 10 minutes, then quickly dip them in cold water for a few seconds. Repeat this process several times.

Chamomile and Daisies

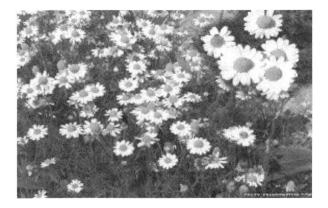

These two natural herbs can be made into an infusion to counter migraines. Perhaps you could go for a leisurely stroll outside the city, somewhere that you can find chamomile and daisies growing naturally. Not only will you benefit from a relaxing walk in nature, but you can also pick these useful ingredients to guard against migraines.

To prepare a brew, place a heaped teaspoon of daisy and chamomile cuttings into a cup of boiling water. Let the blend infuse for one minute. We recommend drinking 2 cups a day.

Linden infusion

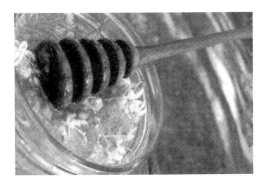

Dried linden is an effective weapon against migraines. When a migraine strikes, take 1.5 tablespoons of linden inflorescence, pour it into 2 cups of boiling water and brew for 15 minutes. Drain the brew.

We recommend drinking ½ a cup of this mixture, 3 times per day.

Lemons

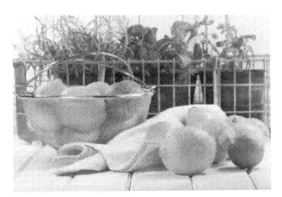

A lemon compress is another way of stopping migraines in their tracks. Squeeze the juice of one lemon and place it in the refrigerator for approximately 10 minutes. Soak a piece of gauze in the chilled juice and then apply to the forehead and temples. Leave it on for half an hour.

Chapter 3: Muscle Pain & Soreness

Usually, my muscle pain is brought about by lack of warming up before working out or overdoing chores around the house and yard. Properly warming up before exercise can help to prevent injury and soreness.

Items on my shelf for Muscle Pain & Soreness:

Epsom Salts: A warm bath in Epsom salts is soothing and detoxifying. Add a little peppermint oil to your bath with the salts to aid in releasing muscle tension.

Peppermint Essential Oil: Rub right onto sore areas. If you have sensitive skin, use a carrier oil like olive oil or coconut oil along with the peppermint oil.

Arnica Gel: Rub in areas that are sore

Arnica Montana: Homeopathic remedy for soreness. Take the recommended dosage.

Meadowsweet pain Elixir

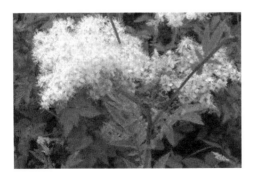

Indications:

This elixir is safe for most individuals, although you may have to use it with caution if you have the flu, chickenpox, or asthma.

Ingredients:

Meadowsweet flowers (100 grams)

Glycerin (100 milliliters)

Vodka, 50-percent (400 milliliters)

Directions:

1. Take a large glass jar and fill with the meadowsweet flowers.

2. Pour the glycerin and vodka into the jar. Shake well to combine everything.

3. Let the mixture stand for one month to six weeks. To ensure that the meadowsweet flowers stay covered by liquid, weigh them down with a weight or a clean stone. You may also add more alcohol to cover the flowers, which gradually absorb the liquid.

4. Pour the mixture through a clean cheesecloth.

5. Transfer the strained mixture into a labeled bottle.

Ginger Fomentation

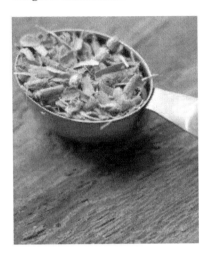

Indications:

This easy-to-make ginger fomentation can ease muscle spasms and menstrual cramps.

Ingredients:

Water (2 cups)

Cramp bark (1/4 cup)

Ginger, dried (1/4 cup)

Cayenne powder (1 tablespoon)

Directions:

1. Fill a pan with the water before adding the cayenne powder and cramp bark.

2. Cover the pan and heat on medium and let simmer for about twenty to thirty minutes.

3. Strain the mixture and then let stand until it is warm to the touch.

4. To use your ginger fomentation, dip a clean washcloth in it. Wring out any excess liquid from the cloth, then place on your affected area. Top the cloth with your hot water bottle before covering with a towel. Allow the fomentation to do its work for about twenty minutes to one hour.

Greaseless Pain Ointment

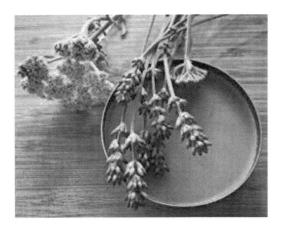

Indications:

Say goodbye to aches, pains, sprains, strains, and bruises with this herbal pain ointment. Apply it several times a day for best results.

Ingredients:

Coconut oil (25 grams)

Infused oil, arnica + St. John's wort (3/4 cup)

Helichrysum hydrosol (2/3 cup)

Shea butter (20 grams)

Lavender essential oil (40 drops)

Beeswax (20 grams)

Directions:

1. In your double boiler place coconut oil, shea butter, and beeswax. Heat the mixture on low to allow the ingredients to melt.

2. Once completely melted, top the mixture with the arnica and St. John's wort infused the oil. Use a popsicle stick to stir everything as you go.

3. Once the beeswax starts to solidify, turn off the double boiler. Stir the mixture again to make sure everything is well-combined. You may reheat the mixture to ensure that the beeswax is completely melted.

4. Pour the melted, still-warm ointment mixture into a food processor or blender. Let the mixture sit until it has adequately cooled and becomes semi-solid.

5. Turn the food processor or blender on before gradually trickling in the coconut oil, lavender essential oil, and helichrysum hydrosol. Stir everything as you go.

6. Before the ointment completely solidifies, transfer into a glass container and store in a cool place.

Cayenne Salve

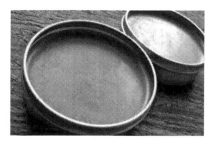

Indications:

Use this homemade cayenne salve on migraine headaches, bruises, arthritis, shingles, backaches, menstrual cramps, and diabetic neuropathy.

Ingredients:

Beeswax (1/2 ounce)

Olive oil (1/2 cup)

Cayenne powder (2 tablespoons)

Directions:

1. Combine the olive oil and cayenne powder by stirring in a small pan heated on medium.

2. Once the mixture is warm, and the cayenne powder is fully incorporated into the olive oil, remove from the heat and let sit for twenty minutes.

3. Do step 3 several times within a twenty-four hour period.

4. Strain the mixture through a clean cheesecloth. Set the infused oil aside.

5. Meanwhile, place the beeswax in a separate pan heated on medium. Once the beeswax has melted, add the infused oil and stir well to combine.

6. Transfer the prepared salve into clean tins or jars. Let cool and label properly.

7. To use your cayenne salve, simply apply it to the affected area. It should only be used in external applications. If using it to treat arthritic pain, use it daily for one to two weeks. If using it to treat hand pain, apply at night and cover with gloves.

Chapter 4: Toothache

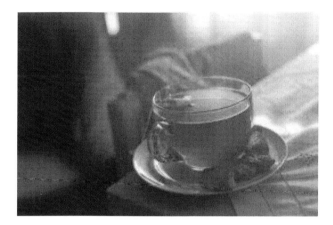

Ingredients

1 tablespoon ground ginger

1 teaspoon ground turmeric

1 pinch black pepper

1 black tea bag

Boil in a mug and enjoy slowly

How to Use:

Tea is a great way to cleanse the body and heal pains from the inside-out. This can be through oral use– you can swish the tea around and focus on the part that is in pain, or you can drink it and allow the warm, healing effect to take place all over your body.

Chapter 5: Colds

Everyone has probably had at least one cold sore in their life. It is very common. However, the reasons for the appearance of such inflammations are varied. It may be caused by yeast infection, allergies, syphilis, and even cancer.

Cold sore caused by allergies is most commonly due to an allergy to nickel. Even more frequently, however, this ailment is caused by yeast.

Cracks at the edges of your lips may also be a sign of a deficiency of vitamin B2 in the body, irritation caused by the dental prosthesis, a reduction in the body's resistance or diabetes.

A properly balanced diet is the best weapon against cold sores. Make sure you consume lots of foods that are sources of B vitamins. Vitamin B2 appears in milk and dairy products, yeast, buckwheat, germ, bran, cereals, tomatoes, green peas, and chives. You should build up your resistance to cold sores, particularly in Autumn and Winter, using be careful with your diet. Garlic is a great natural way to increase immunity and also it offers bactericidal activity.

Lemon Tea or Raspberry Juice

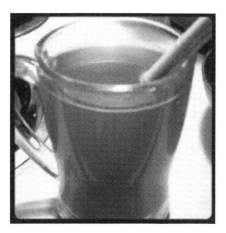

Lemon and the homemade raspberry juice tastes great with hot tea, which effectively quenches thirst. This mixture makes the body warms up and sweat. Raspberry juice can be prepared simply and the homemade version is more effective than the one you can buy from the shop.

The recipe for raspberry juice comprises 1 kg of raspberries and 20 grams of sugar.

Clean the raspberries and put them in a pot. Pour in a little water, then add 10 grams of sugar, then cook. When the fruit is cooked, separate the pulp from the raspberries through a sieve. Sweeten the juice according to tastes, then bring it to boil again and pour into jars. Once cooled, store in a cold place and consume when you have a cold or feel one coming on.

Vitamin C

Vitamin C, also called ascorbic acid, has a strong antiviral impact. A deficiency in vitamin C can cause the common cold, so you need to remember to take it, but not necessarily in pill form. Instead, it's easy to get the required amount of vitamin C in fruit and vegetables, such as broccoli, spinach, potatoes, apples, oranges, grapefruits, lemons, kiwi, cabbage, cauliflower, peppers, artichokes, tomatoes, melons, and pineapples.

Antibacterial Garlic

Garlic is a key weapon in fighting colds because it has antibacterial properties. Sometimes people are wary of using this remedy because of the garlic's odor. If you can't face swallowing even a little of this natural medicine, you can instead crush a clove of garlic and then inhale the 'aroma.'

Moisturizing Stuffy Nose

Having a stuffy or blocked nose makes it difficult to breathe properly, so we must take care of mucosal hydration. Make sure you have a lot to drink, and above all, keep the air around you wet. Lay wet towels on radiators and keep all rooms in your house airy.

Sore, Cracked Skin

Everyone knows the uncomfortable feeling when the skin around the nose because sore and cracked while suffering from a cold. You can alleviate this by using calendula ointment, which will make you feel relieved and help the skin regenerate faster.

Camphor Oil

This is a great remedy for a sore throat and stuffy nose. Simply rub the camphor oil around your neck, keeping its place with a warm scarf or dressing. This keeps the throat is hot and helps you to easily breathe through your nose.

Bath

Taking a bath before bed, you also help to get rid of a fever. Lie in warm water for about 10 minutes. Make sure the water temperature is not lower than 2 ° C of your body temperature. Otherwise, the bath may only be harmful and won't help.

If you find that these home remedies for colds do not help and symptoms persist, make sure you see a doctor without delay.

Milk With Honey

Drinking warm milk is a common solution for cold-related symptoms, but adding honey makes it so much better. Even though honey lacks vitamins, it does effectively get rid of bacteria. It can have positive effects in the alleviation of a strong cough.

If you have a fever or a headache (or both!), soak a towel in cold water and then put it on your forehead and chest. To make it even cooler, wrap ice in the towel. Your temperature will decrease, and your head will stop hurting. Don't cool the body for any longer than 15 minutes.

Sage and Chamomile

The infusion of sage and chamomile is not particularly tasty. It is, however, very helpful for sore throats because it acts as an antibiotic. Place a spoonful of the sage and chamomile in a cup, then pour in boiling water. Leave the mixture covered for about 10 minutes, drain and then rinse down the throat. For the best results, do so at least 3 times a day for several days.

Chapter 6: Runny Nose

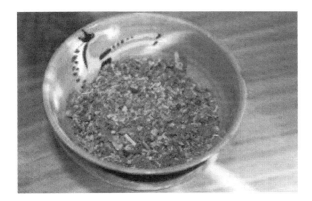

A runny nose is the plague of the winter season. This ailment is all too well known and can impede daily functioning. So how do we fight this and quickly get back to enjoying good health?

Many factors can cause a runny nose. It is usually a viral infection, but it this is not the only cause. It may be the result of an allergic reaction or inflammation of the sinuses. Here is what distinguishes this variety of ailments, also known as rhinitis:

Bacterial infection

This may be due to excess nasal mucosa, which can be caused by previous virus infections.

Viruses

This most common variety can occur at any time of the year, but mostly it occurs when the body has a reduced resistance, namely in Autumn and Winter.

Allergies

Pollen most often causes this type of rhinitis. It is sometimes known as hay fever and usually occurs during Spring.

The symptoms of such an infection include:

A stuffy or blocked nose.

Difficulty in breathing.

Numbness, an inability to recognize odors or flavors.

Headaches.

Watery eyes.

Loss or reduction in appetite.

Fever.

Visible inflammation, redness of the nose.

Itchy nose.

Frequent sneezing.

Vitamin C

An effective way of reducing the symptoms is to eat a lot of hot (until steaming) meals and drinking many of warm fluids, such as tea with lemon juice, or elderflower. Add garlic to your meals. Eat plenty of fruit (oranges, apples), which are rich in the natural and most absorbable forms of vitamins.

Everyone knows about the miraculous attributes of Vitamin C. Taking this popular tablet 2 or 3 times per day may speed up our recovery from a cold. You can also try soluble tablets, in the form of hot fluid. Drink and eat hot!

Chapter 7: Sore Throat & Coughs

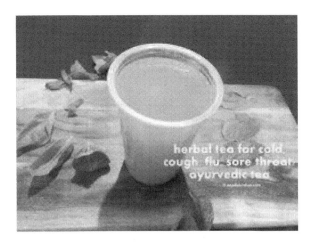

A sore throat is just painful and annoying. A virus causes the majority of sore throats, so antibiotics would not aid in healing. Warm beverages and keeping the throat moist with steam treatments can give relief.

Items on my shelf for Sore Throats:

Eucalyptus Essential Oil: Use the steam method as described for colds. Place a cup of mullein leaves and 3-4 cups of water in a pot and bring to a boil. After it comes to a boil, add 2-3 drops of eucalyptus oil, and drape a towel over your head. Inhale the steam. Be careful, as the liquid is very hot.

Sea Salt: Gargle with sea salt and warm water.

Apple Cider Vinegar: Drink 1 teaspoon with 8 ounces of water. Gargle with ACV and water.

Raw Honey: Take a teaspoon of Raw Honey

Cough Drops: Ricola Natural Herb Cough Drops are a favorite to tame a cough when you are away from home.

Homemade Cough Syrups

1. Chocolate Syrup

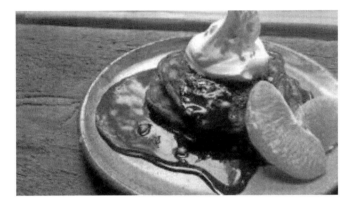

Not only is this effective at relieving coughs, but it also tastes delicious. You'll have no problem getting your children to take it.

You will need:

- 4 Tablespoons honey.

- 1 Tablespoon Apple cider vinegar.

- 3 tablespoons water.

- 4 tablespoons melted chocolate; preferably dark chocolate.

- ¼ teaspoon grated ginger; preferably fresh ginger.

- ½ teaspoon grated garlic; preferably fresh.

- Pinch of cayenne pepper

This is another mixture which is very easy to make. Simply place all the ingredients into a sealable jar or container and shake vigorously for several minutes.

2. Olive Cough Syrup

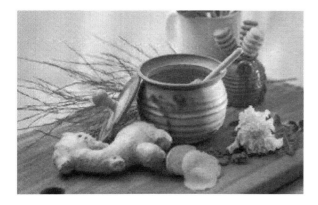

You will need:

- 1 Cup liquid honey.

- ½ cup olive oil.

- 1 freshly squeezed lemon.

Mixing them is easy; you simply need a suitably sized container and then place all the ingredients into it. Shake vigorously until they are fully blended and then store the syrup in the refrigerator.

3. Ginger & Pepper

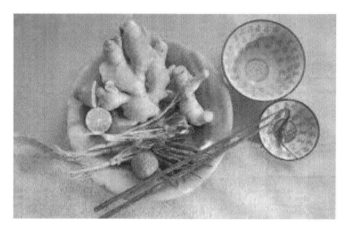

Keep it simple with this easy and effective syrup recipe:

You will need:

- 1 cup of warm water.

- 2 tablespoons Dried ginger.

- 2 tablespoons dried Thyme.

- 2 tablespoons dried black pepper.

- 12 tablespoons of honey.

Start by mixing the honey and the warm water. This can be warm from the tap or heated gently in the microwave or on the stove.

Next slowly add the ginger, thyme, and pepper. Stir it well as you do so. The mixture will become syrup. You lay prefer to whisk your mixture to ensue it is blended thoroughly.

You can then store it in a sealed container. If you keep it in a cool place away from direct sunlight, it should last for three or four weeks.

Take one teaspoon as and when you need it; there is no limit regarding how many times a day you can take this syrup.

4. Ginger Syrup

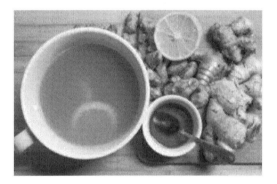

You'll need:

- 1tsp of ground ginger

- A pinch of cayenne pepper

- 3 tablespoons Honey, preferably runny honey.

- 3 tablespoons apple cider vinegar

- 1 lemon juiced

- 1 cup of water.

Making this remedy is simple! All you need to do is place all the ingredients inside a bottle or container which can be sealed shut.

The mixture should be kept in a sealed container, but it does not need to be kept in the refrigerator.

Chapter 8: Diarrhea

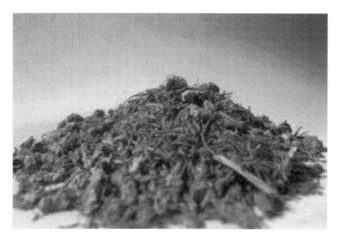

This is an unpleasant but common illness that affects everyone at some point in their life. While the cause may not always be known, there is a good chance that it is from a mild infection which will quickly clear by itself.

However, you need to do something about diarrhea!

Try one of these herbal antibiotics:

Goldenseal

Goldenseal is recognized as being a powerful natural herbal antibiotic. It is used to help cancer patients.

The key ingredient in this herb is berberine which is known to be antimicrobial, anti-inflammatory and can even lower your blood glucose levels. It also improves the flow of food and drinks through your digestive tract; reducing the likelihood of bacteria collecting and preventing diarrhea.

Add 40 drops of the liquid herbal extracts to a small glass of water. You should do this 3 times a day.

Of course, you can harvest the roots of this plant and dry them to make your tea.

Astragalus

This powerful herb is known to have polysaccharides; these help your immune system to fight off diseases. It is also antiviral and antibacterial which will assist you in dealing with any infection, quickly stopping the issue which is causing you to have diarrhea.

This is another herb which can be turned into tea, and this is very effective when dealing with diarrhea. It adds water to your body and surprisingly diarrhea can cause you to dehydrate fast.

Simply boil 5g of the dried root powder in 12 ounces of water. Ideally, you should drink this three times every day to boost your immune system and prevent diarrhea before it even happens!

Chapter 9: Intestinal Problems

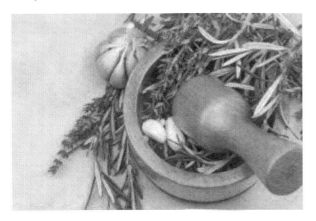

You've probably experienced that pain in your stomach before and wondered whether you have simply got trapped wind or something more serious. Whether you have heartburn or stomach cramps, the pain can be unbearable. IBS is one of the most common issues which can, fortunately, be helped with these antibiotic herbs:

Ginger

This herb also makes a reappearance, proving how powerful its antibiotic effects are.

Ginger is known to alleviate nausea and sooth the digestive process.

Ginger can be consumed in your meals or be used to make tea. You can even boil sliced ginger root in water with a little sugar to make a drink. Whether you dilute it with water o not will depend upon your tastes.

It is worth noting that too much ginger can cause stomach upsets. However this is in large doses, a few grams a day will help your system.

Turmeric

This powerful herb makes another appearance in the book as it is known to help with liver function and aid the digestive process.

The best way to take turmeric is to add a teaspoon of the dried powder to your food each day.

Chapter 10: Acne

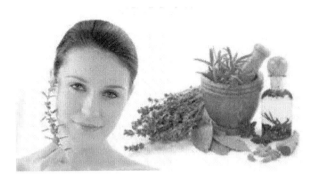

Acne is something that most people associate with their teenage years as it is directly linked to the surge of hormones in that period of your life.

Yeast

The first answer to conversations about remedies for acne is of course yeast. This can be applied to a few different methods:

Drinking

Add ¼ of a cube of yeast to warm milk and wait for it to dissolve. The milk can also be at room temperature if desired. Prepare this drink for yourself once a day. This will help to noticeably reduce your acne, and also result in a general improvement to the health of your skin.

Mask

This is a reliable method that can be used regularly. Wash and dry your face thoroughly. Then apply a slurry of yeast that has been dissolved in a small amount of milk and a few drops of olive oil. Leave the solution on your face for approximately 20 minutes. Then, wash the mask off your face using warm, preferably boiled water.

If you want to have the highest possible impact, do this treatment once per week at least. Yeast is great for the skin and so is a suitable treatment for acne.

Home tonics

Some special home tonics can be used to eradicate acne. Try these out!

Aloe

We've already discussed the use of aloe for herpes, but it's also useful in the treatment of acne. You can use aloe to wash acne-infected skin or use its aqueous solution. Aloe juice can be bought directly from a pharmacy or drained from the actual plant leaves if you feel like purchasing from a florist or nursery. Aloe extract is a common ingredient in many cosmetics that are specifically formulated for sensitive or juvenile acne-prone skin. That should be evidence enough that it is an effective anti-acne weapon!

Cucumber

Cucumber is very soothing on the skin. It also tapers pores and has a moisturizing effect. Add grated cucumber to boiled or bottled water. Take note that the juice should not be withdrawn. Apply the mixture to the acne with a cotton swab.

Lemon

Add a few drops of lemon juice to a large bowl of previously boiled water. You can also use bottled or spring water. Soak a cotton swab in the resulting tonic and use it to wash the affected area. Because of its disinfectant properties, lemon can help to brighten and nourish your skin, and of course, get rid of that acne.

However, acne can reappear at any stage of your life and can cause embarrassment or even restrict you from completing certain activities.

Basil

They are two types of Basil, Holy and Sweet but they are both effective against acne. You have two options:

Sweet Basil is excellent when mixed with coconut oil. Simply add equal measures of both and blend then apply it directly to your skin. You'll dry out the spot and hydrate the skin in one go.

Holy basil can be made into a tea by placing ten leaves of the plant into a cup of boiling water and allowing it to brew for 5 minutes. This tea will help to balance your hormones; preventing further outbreaks.

Cinnamon Spot Treatment

Take one tablespoon of cinnamon and mix it with a few drops of honey, it should be just enough to make a paste. Then mix in a pinch of nutmeg.

Whenever a spot appears to apply some of this directly to it for up to 2 hours. The natural antibiotics in cinnamon will kill the bacteria in the spot while the honey and the nutmeg replenish the skin. You'll be surprised at the results!

Conclusion

I hope this book was able to help you to realize that preparing your herbal remedies at home does not have to be a science experiment. Hopefully, this book has shown you that it is possible to treat your family with homemade herbal medicine. Then you will be prepared to turn to a natural remedy at a moment's notice.

Please remember that this book is not an exhaustive resource since the world of natural remedies is so vast. I encourage you that if you are spurred on to learn more, do some research, and see what remedies work best for your family.

The next step is to take your time experimenting with the recipes provided in this book.

Made in the USA
Middletown, DE
20 September 2023

38914207R00024